A Remedy for Obesity

(How to Stop Obsessing About Food and Lose Weight an Antidote to Obesity)

William E. Guillory

Chapter 1

Introduction:

Chapter 1

INTRODUCTION

 for Obesity: How to Stop Obsessing About Food and Lose Weight The Antidote to Obesity is a book that offers a solution to the growing problem of obesity. The book begins by discussing the causes of obesity, including our modern lifestyle and diet. It then provides a step-by-step guide to overcoming these factors and losing weight in a healthy and sustainable way. The book also provides tips for changing one's mindset and habits to support long-term weight loss. Finally, it offers recipes and meal plans to help readers put the book's advice into practice.

The book starts by exploring the biological and psychological factors that contribute to obesity. It explains how our modern lifestyles and diets, full of processed and high-calorie foods, can result in gaining weight. The effects of stress and sleep deprivation on weight are also covered in the book. The book then offers a comprehensive strategy for weight loss that incorporates exercise, a healthy diet, and a positive outlook. It highlights the importance of small changes over time rather than quick fixes or fad diets.

One of the key concepts in the book is "mindful eating." This involves paying attention to what, when, and how we eat, rather than just eating mindlessly. The book provides strategies for tuning into our hunger and fullness cues and making better food choices. The book also offers a 10-week plan for making changes and reaching weight-loss goals. This plan includes tips for meal planning, grocery shopping, cooking, and enjoying meals without overeating. The book also provides recipes and ideas for healthy meals that are both satisfying and nutritious.

A Remedy for Obesity: How to Stop Obsessing About Food and Lose Weight is a good choice if you're looking for a book to aid in weight loss. It's a wise decision to use the antidote to obesity. The book offers a sensible, long-term strategy for weight loss. Instead of quick fixes or fad diets, it places an emphasis on lifestyle changes and healthy habits. Additionally, it provides a 10-week strategy for implementing the book's recommendations. This book can assist you in achieving your weight loss objectives in a sustainable and healthy manner, with a focus on mindful eating. Click the **buy button** right away.

Chapter 1

The Obesity Epidemic and the Need for a Long-Term Solution

The significant and ongoing rise in the prevalence of obesity within a population over time is referred to as an "obesity epidemic." A high body mass index (BMI) is typically used to define obesity, which has emerged as a major global health issue.
The obesity epidemic is a significant issue that requires attention. Nearly 40% of adults in the US are obese, and this number is steadily increasing, according to the CDC. Obesity is linked to a number of serious medical conditions, including diabetes, heart disease, and some cancers. And it's a problem that

affects the entire world, not just the United States.

However, how do we fix it? There is no simple solution, but I believe a mix of community outreach, policy changes, and education is the key

simply don't know how to make healthy choices. They may not have access to healthy foods, or they may not know how to cook healthy meals. We need to educate people about nutrition and provide them with the resources they need to make healthy choices. That includes everything from cooking classes to food subsidies for low-income families. And then there's the issue of policy.

We need to change our food environment so that it's easier to make healthy choices. That means things like improving the nutritional standards for school lunches and providing incentives for restaurants to offer healthier options.

. **Health Consequences**: Obesity is linked to a variety of health issues. These can include an increased risk of cardiovascular disease, stroke, type 2 diabetes, certain cancers, and musculoskeletal disorders. It can also result in a lower quality of life and higher healthcare costs.

Poor dietary choices, sedentary lifestyles, genetics, socioeconomic status, access to healthy foods, and environmental factors such as the availability of safe places to exercise are all factors.

Short-Term vs. Long-Term Solutions: Short-term obesity solutions frequently involve rapid weight loss through methods such as crash diets, which may not be sustainable and can result in weight regain. Long-term solutions emphasise making long-term lifestyle changes, such as eating a balanced diet and exercising regularly, to maintain a healthy weight over time.

Importance for Public Health:

Addressing the obesity epidemic is critical for public health. Obesity's high prevalence strains healthcare systems by increasing demand for medical services to treat obesity-related health issues. It also has an impact on economic productivity and general well-being.

The following is the purpose of the article or presentation:

The article's or presentation's purpose may differ. It could aim to raise awareness about the obesity epidemic, educate the public about its causes and consequences, propose strategies for dealing with it on an individual or societal level, or advocate for policy changes to encourage healthier lifestyles.

These topics are frequently discussed in the introduction to provide context and set the stage for the main content of the article or presentation, which may go into greater

depth, solutions
research findings, and recommendations.

Chapter 2

Definition of Obesity:

An excessive amount of body fat characterises obesity, a medical condition. Body mass index (BMI) is a measurement that is frequently used to define it. The square of a person's height in metres divided by their weight in kilogrammes yields their BMI. Obesity is typically defined as having a BMI of 30 or higher. Typical BMI classifications include

A BMI less than 18.5 indicates underweight. BMI of 18.5 to 24.9 for a healthy weight BMI 25 to 29.9 for overweight Obese: BMI of 30 or higher It's crucial to remember that BMI has its limitations and cannot take into account elements like muscle mass, bone density, and fat distribution. As a result, it might not give a full picture of a person's health.

There isn't a single, obvious reason why people become obese. It is a multifactorial condition affected by a wide range of connected factors.

Dietary Practises: Unhealthy eating habits like overindulging in high-calorie, low-nutrient foods (commonly referred to as "junk food"), drinking sugary beverages, and eating a lot of food all at once cause weight gain and obesity. Processed food and added sugar-heavy diets are particularly harmful.

Sedentary lifestyles: Sedentary behaviours, such as spending extended periods of time sitting still and getting little exercise, can result in weight gain. This factor is influenced by contemporary lifestyles that include desk jobs, screen time, and little physical activity.

Genetics: Although there is some genetic component to obesity, it is not the only factor. Some people may be genetically predisposed to obesity, which makes it easier for them.

Environmental Factors: The built environment and community design can either support or hinder healthy choices. Some people are genetically predisposed to obesity, which makes it easier for them.

Emotional and Psychological Factors: Emotional eating, stress, depression, and other psychological factors can cause overeating and contribute to obesity, for instance, in neighbourhoods without access to fresh produce or secure parks.

Social and cultural norms: Eating habits can be influenced by cultural customs and societal expectations. Large, calorie-dense meals are frequently served at celebratory events, and social pressure can make people overeat. Hormonal imbalances, including those that encourage weight gain, can result from some medical conditions and medications. Examples include hypothyroidism or polycystic ovary syndrome (PCOS) conditions.

There isn't just one clear reason why people get fat. It is a multifactorial condition that is influenced by many interrelated factors.

Dietary Guidelines: Weight gain and obesity are brought on by unhealthy eating patterns like bingeing on high-calorie, low-nutrient foods (commonly referred to as "junk food"), drinking sugary beverages, and eating a lot of food at once. Diets high in processed food and added sugar are particularly harmful. Sedentary lifestyles can lead to weight gain because they involve spending a lot of time sitting still and getting little exercise. Modern lifestyles, which include desk jobs, screen time, and little physical activity, have an impact on

Genetics: Obesity does have a genetic component, but it is not the only one. Some individuals might have genetic

Identifying these causes is crucial for creating efficient obesity prevention plans. Promoting healthy eating practices, encouraging physical activity, and creating environments that support these decisions are just a few of the interventions that are frequently needed to address obesity. It's also crucial to take into account how individualised obesity is, as a person's solution may not be the same as another's due to the influence of genetic and environmental factors.

chapter 3

In "The psychological Aspect of Food Obsession and Emotional Eating

 the emotional and psychological triggers for food obsession and binge eating, particularly when triggered by emotions, are examined. It explores the complex interplay between our feelings, thoughts, and

can help people with food obsessions deal with the underlying causes and establish healthier relationships with food and their bodies.

Constant Food Thoughts: People who are food-obsessed may discover that their daily lives are dominated by food-related thoughts. They might constantly consider their next opportunity to eat, obsessively plan meals, and track their caloric intake. Food Obsession and Compulsive Eating: People who are food obsessed may develop compulsive eating, where they feel compelled to eat a lot of food frequently.

This behaviour may result in binge eating and a loss of self-control. Some people may use food as their main source of comfort to deal with stress, sadness, or other emotions. This is known as an emotional attachment to food.

They might use food as a coping mechanism for their emotional distress. Unhealthy Relationship with Food: Obsession with food can lead to an unhealthy relationship with food, where people label foods as "good" or "bad," which causes them to feel guilty or anxious when they eat. Body Image Concerns:

People who are obsessed with their appearance and think that strict diet control is required to attain or maintain an ideal body shape are oftentimes linked to food obsessions.

Social Isolation: People who suffer from a severe food obsession may distance themselves from social events and get-togethers in order to stay away from situations that entail food. Their quality of life may suffer as a result, and they may become socially isolated.

Extreme food obsessions can lead to the development of eating disorders, including binge eating disorder, bulimia nervosa, and anorexia nervosa.

An obsession with food, also known as a food preoccupation or obsession, is a condition in which a person's thoughts and actions around food become unhealthy and all-consuming. **This obsession with food can take many**

 1 obsession of Food: People who are obsessed with food may find that their daily lives are dominated by thoughts about food. They might count calories, plan meals inordinately, and obsessively consider when they will get to eat again.

2. **Compulsive Eating:** Obsession with food can result in compulsive eating, a condition in which a person feels compelled to eat a lot of food, frequently and quickly. This kind of behaviour can result in binge eating and a loss of self-control.

3. **Food-Related Emotions:** Some people may turn to food as their main comfort, turning to it to help them deal with stress, grief, or other emotions. They might use food as a coping mechanism for their emotional distress.

4. **Unhealthy Relationship with Food:** Obsession with food can lead to an unhealthy

relationship with food, where people label foods as "good" or "bad," which causes them to feel guilty and anxious when they eat.

5 Personal Image Issues: Food obsession is frequently associated with problems with body image, as people become fixated on their appearance and think that maintaining or achieving an ideal body shape requires strict dietary control.

6. Social Detachment: In extreme circumstances, anorexics may distance themselves from social events and get-togethers in order to avoid situations involving food. Their quality of life may suffer as a result, and they may become socially isolated.

7. Eating Illnesses: In severe circumstances, an obsession with food may play a role in the emergence of eating disorders like bulimia nervosa, anorexia nervosa, or binge eating disorder.

Of course, let's take a closer look at the methods for overcoming emotional eating:

 1. Identifying the Triggers: To record when and why you eat, keep a journal. Make a note of the feelings, circumstances, or occurrences that make you want to eat. You can better understand what triggers emotional eating by recognising patterns.

2. Intentional Consumption:

Take great note of the eating process. Eat without being distracted by electronics like the TV, computer, or phone. Enjoy every bite and stay in the present. This improves your awareness of your body's signals of hunger and fullness.

3. Emotion Recognition: Acquire the ability to recognise and categorise your feelings. Consider whether the urge to eat is an emotional reaction or a physical hunger when you get it. One of the most important first steps in treating emotional eating is realising your feelings.

5. **Organise Healthy Snacks:** If you are aware that you often eat when you are upset, keep wholesome snacks close at hand. These could include things like yoghurt, fruits, vegetables, or a small amount of nuts. Nutritious snack choices help curb cravings without encouraging overindulgence.

6. Maintain Hydration:

Feelings of hunger can occasionally be brought on by dehydration. Make sure you stay hydrated throughout the day by drinking enough water. Have a glass of water first if you're not sure if you're hungry or thirsty.

7. Steer clear of restrictive diets: Overly stringent dietary guidelines and severe dieting can raise the risk of emotional eating. Rather, concentrate on sustainable, well-balanced eating practices that let you indulge in a large range of foods in moderation.

 8. Practice Portion Control: Use portion control if you choose to eat out of emotion. Measure out a sensible portion and save it slowly, rather than mindlessly devouring the entire bag of snacks.

9. **Ask for Help:**

You might want to talk to a support group, therapist, or counsellor about your emotional eating patterns. They can offer helpful advice and coping mechanisms to deal with the underlying emotional problems that trigger emotional eating.

10. **Remain Active:** Getting regular exercise helps reduce stress and elevate mood. Exercise can assist in lowering the emotional appetite for food. Aim for 150 minutes or more a week of moderate-to-intense aerobic exercise.

Keep in mind that beating emotional eating is a process that takes time, and it's acceptable to experience setbacks.

The secret is to practice self-compassion and concentrate on transforming your relationship with food and emotions in a way that will last. If your everyday life and well-being are greatly affected by emotional eating, it may be especially helpful to seek professional assistance. Effective comprehension and management of the underlying emotional issues can be aided by a therapist or counsellor.

It's crucial to remember that a food obsession may indicate deeper emotional or psychological problems. People who struggle with food obsession may find it helpful to seek assistance from a mental health professional, such as a therapist or counsellor, in order to address the underlying causes and create healthier relationships with food and their bodies.

Chapter 4

Mindful Eating, a Balanced Diet, and Developing a Positive Relationship with Food

To make sure your body gets all the vital nutrients it needs, a balanced diet consists of a variety of foods. The following recommendations will assist you in achieving a balanced diet: Keep in mind that every person has different nutritional needs, so it's critical to customise your diet to your particular needs and preferences. Your body gets the nutrients it needs for optimum health and wellbeing from a balanced diet.

Fruits and Vegetables: Try to include a range of vibrant fruits and vegetables to fill half of your plate. They supply vital minerals, vitamins, and fibre.

Lean protein sources such as fish, poultry, beans, tofu, and lean meat cuts should be included in your diet. Protein is essential for healthy muscles, tissue growth, and general wellbeing.

Whole Grains: Refined grains are not as good as whole grains. For complex carbs and fibre, choose whole wheat, brown rice, quinoa, and oats. Healthy Fats: Include foods high in unsaturated fats, like olive oil, almonds, seeds, and avocados. For general health and heart health, these fats are essential.

Dairy or Dairy Alternatives: Select low-fat or fat-free dairy products if you eat them. If you don't tolerate lactose or would rather use a substitute, you might want to look into soy, almond, or coconut milk.

Reduce Added Sugars: Pay attention to the added sugars in processed meals and sugar-filled drinks. Reduce the amount you consume to lower your chance of health issues.

Protein Control: Be mindful of portion sizes to prevent overindulgence. This is where smaller plates come in handy.

Hydration: To stay hydrated, sip lots of water throughout the day. Thirst can occasionally be confused with hunger.

Meal Timing: To sustain energy levels and avoid overindulging, try spreading meals and snacks out throughout the day.

Balanced Snacks: To keep yourself full in between meals, choose healthy snacks like Greek yoghurt, almonds, or fresh fruit.

Plan Ahead: By organising your meals ahead of time, you can steer clear of impulsive, less nourishing options and make healthier decisions.

Moderation: Balance calls for a variety of foods, but moderation is also a part of that. Savour sweets and indulgences with awareness.

Speak with an Expert: Consider seeking individualised advice from a registered dietitian or nutritionist if you have particular dietary requirements or health concerns.

It takes time and self-compassion to develop a positive relationship with food. It's about taking care of your body, appreciating food, and realising that your general state of health is not defined by any one meal or snack. Mix up your diet by including a variety of foods from every dietary group. This keeps your diet from becoming monotonous and guarantees that you get a wide range of nutrients.

 Portion Control: Consider the size of your portions. To help you manage portion sizes, use smaller plates and pay attention to your body's signals of hunger and fullness.

Nutrient-Dense Foods: Give special attention to foods high in nutrients, such as fruits, vegetables, whole grains, lean proteins, and healthy fats. These supply vital minerals and vitamins.

Hydration: Throughout the day, sip a lot of water. Thirst can occasionally be confused with hunger.

Mindful Eating: Be mindful of the food you're consuming. When dining, keep your eyes off of screens like TVs and cell phones and enjoy the flavours and textures of your food.

Harmony Aim for a balanced proportion of macronutrients, including proteins, fats, and carbohydrates. In your diet, fats, proteins, and carbohydrates are all essential.

Treats should be enjoyed in moderation. A balanced diet allows for the occasional indulgence, but it shouldn't control your entire eating schedule.

Typical Meals: Consume regular meals and snacks to keep your energy up and avoid overindulging when you're really hungry.

Take Note of Your Body: Observe your body's signals of hunger and fullness. When you're hungry, eat, and when you're satisfied, stop.

Make a plan. To help you make healthier decisions, schedule your meals and snacks in advance.

Avert Emotional Eating: Look for non-food solutions to handle tension or feelings. Unhealthy food relationships can result from emotional eating.

Speak with an expert Consult a qualified dietitian or nutritionist

Chapter 5

Exercise and Physical Activity: Choosing an Interest: Including Movement in Everyday Life

Physical activity and exercise; selecting a hobby; including movement in daily life Physical activity and exercise are essential for losing weight and enhancing general health. Because fat loss is a gradual process, it's critical to combine exercise with a healthy diet and lifestyle. Here are some tips to help you burn fat through exercise effectively. Furthermore, remember that every person's body reacts to exercise differently, so persevere and be patient with yourself.

Cardiovascular Exercise: Include brisk walking, cycling, swimming, or running as part of your routine. Engaging in these activities can help you lose body fat because they raise your heart rate and burn calories.

High-intensity interval training, or HIIT, alternates short bursts of vigorous exercise with rest intervals in between. It's a powerful method for increasing metabolism and burning fat. Strength Training: Use weights or bodyweight exercises for resistance training. Gaining lean muscle mass can help you burn more calories at rest by raising your resting metabolic rate.

Exercises with Compounds: Pay special attention to exercises with compound movements, such as push-ups, deadlifts, and squats. By using several muscle groups, these exercises increase the number of calories burned.

Core Work: Use exercises like planks and

Russian twists to strengthen your core muscles. In addition to supporting general fat loss, a strong core can enhance posture.

Flexibility and Mobility: Remember to include stretches and exercises that improve flexibility, such as Pilates or yoga. They lessen the chance of injury and increase range of motion.

 Consistency: Include exercise on a daily basis in your schedule. To see long-term benefits from fat loss, consistency is essential.

Progressive Overload: Build up the difficulty and intensity of your exercises gradually. This puts your body to the test and promotes fat loss.

Diet: For fat loss, a balanced diet is enhanced by exercise. Steer clear of unhealthy food choices as an overcompensation for your exercise.

Sufficient Sleep: Obtain enough restorative sleep, as it is essential for controlling hunger hormones and promoting weight loss.

Keep Yourself Hydrated: Good hydration is essential for metabolism and general well-being. Before, during, and after your workouts, sip water.

Track Your Progress: Maintain a log of your exercises and advancement. This can inspire you and assist you in modifying your workout regimen as necessary.

Seek Professional Advice: To develop a customised exercise programme that meets your needs and goals, think about consulting a personal trainer or fitness specialist.

Safety First: Don't overstrain and listen to your body's cues. Should you have any underlying health concerns, seek advice from a healthcare provider.

It is possible to make incorporating

movement into daily life simple, easy, and enjoyable. It doesn't have to be a chore or feel like "exercise" to be effective. It could be anything from doing some light yoga or stretching to going for a stroll in the park. Finding hobbies that suit your lifestyle and that you enjoy is the key. Here are a few recommendations:

Whenever feasible, choose to walk or cycle rather than drive or use public transport.

 Take the stairs rather than the lift. In the morning or evening, try some gentle yoga or stretching.

Adding quick bursts of movement to long stretches of sitting is another way to make movement a part of your life. All it takes to do this is to simply get up from your desk once an hour and take a short stroll. Alternatively, if you work from home, consider taking a break to clean the dishes or run a hoover. Your circulation and energy levels can be improved even if you just stand up and stretch your legs.

You can also try to find ways to incorporate exercise into your free time.

For instance, you could go swimming or hiking rather than just lounging on the couch and watching TV.
It can be entertaining and social to look for opportunities to move your body. You might try playing with your children or pets, signing up for a sports team, or taking a dance class.
It all comes down to figuring out what works for you and incorporating it into your daily routine. And never forget that every little movement matters.
Engaging in physical activity for even ten minutes can improve your health and wellness.
Remember, though, that you don't have to go overboard. As you get fitter and more confident, start out small and increase the amount of movement gradually.

Chapter 6

Recipes and Meal Plans for Long-Term Weight Loss - Delicious and Nutritious Meal Ideas

Plans: Yummy and Healthy Dinner Suggestions

Let's begin with some advice on eating healthily!

Begin by consuming five servings or more of fruits and vegetables each day. They are a good source of fibre, vitamins, and minerals.

Give priority to whole foods, such as lots of fruits and vegetables, lean protein, whole grains, and healthy fats.

Limit sugary drinks, alcohol, and high-fat foods, and drink lots of water.

A Comprehensive Guide to Long-Term Weight Loss:

Recipes and Meal Plans There are a few considerations to make with recipes and meal plans.

First, diversity is essential.

Secondly, attempt to schedule your snacks and meals ahead of time. This can assist you in avoiding making poor decisions when you're famished or in a hurry.

Thirdly, make an effort to prepare more meals at home. This will enable you to manage the amounts and ingredients. It's also typically less expensive and healthier than eating out.

Here are some specific meal ideas to get you going:

Oats, chia seeds, almond milk, and berries are combined to make overnight oats.

A straightforward salad with avocado, tomatoes, cucumbers, and mixed greens dressed with a lemon vinaigrette Quinoa, roasted sweet potatoes, black beans, and Greek yoghurt are combined in a bowl. grilled chicken breast served over sweet potatoes and roasted broccoli.

A vegetable wrap composed of spinach, cucumbers, tomatoes, hummus, avocado, and whole-wheat tortilla a frozen fruit, chia seeds, and unsweetened almond milk smoothie. As you can see, there are lots of delectable and healthy options available. Online resources offer a plethora of additional recipes and meal ideas.

The next action is to concentrate on portion management. Even when you're eating healthy foods, it's easy to overindulge. Being aware of how much you eat and making sure you're not overindulging are key components of portion control. Using smaller plates and bowls is one way to control portion sizes. By doing this, you can prevent overeating and piling food on your plate.
Eat mindfully, taking note of your body's signals of hunger and fullness.

Give yourself time to feel satisfied by pausing in between bites.
The timing of meals is another important component of a healthy diet. Regular eating can help control blood sugar levels and provide you with sustained energy and satisfaction throughout the day. The following advice relates to meal timing:
Within an hour of waking up, start your day with a nutritious breakfast.

Have a little snack every couple of hours.
Try to eat your largest meal during the noon hour.
Consume your final meal of the day two to three hours prior to going to bed.
Steer clear of late-night eating. Sleep disturbances like this can cause you to overeat.

Making the right decisions and eating at the appropriate times are key components of healthy eating. These easy rules will help you eat in a way that is both healthy and pleasurable. It's about making tiny adjustments that add up over time, not about being flawless. So enjoy the journey to a healthier you, and try not to be too hard on yourself.

Chapter 7

Maintaining Your Achievement Strategies for Long-Term Success

Sustaining Your Success Techniques for Extended Periods of Time

Well done on achieving your objectives! Once you've accomplished your goals, the next thing to do is to sustain your success over time. Here are some helpful strategies:

Make new plans. It's time to set new goals now that you've accomplished your original ones. This will support your continued growth and motivation.

Give yourself a treat. Honour your efforts and treat yourself to a reward for your achievements. This will support your motivation and help you stay on course.

Be ready for obstacles. Being unprepared for setbacks is vital because they are an inevitable part of life. Do not give up if you encounter a setback. Refocus instead, and modify your plan as necessary.

Form wholesome routines. Developing wholesome routines that you can stick to is one of the best ways to maintain your accomplishments. For instance, if you've been working out frequently,

Exercise a few times a week as a habit. Make it a habit to prepare healthy meals at home if you've been eating a balanced diet.

Seek assistance. Having a solid support network is essential to sustaining your accomplishments. Those who will support and encourage you on your journey should be in your immediate vicinity. This could be a support group, family, or friends.

Remain optimistic. Sustaining an optimistic outlook is crucial for sustained achievement. Maintain a growth mindset and stay in the present. Recall that the objective is progress, not perfection.

You can sustain your accomplishments over time and stay on course by using these tactics.

Always exercise patience and proceed cautiously. You can do this!

Maintaining your accomplishments also requires you to prioritise self-care. This entails looking after your mental, emotional, and physical well-being.

Make sure you're eating a balanced diet, getting enough sleep, and exercising for your physical well-being. Try to manage your stress and engage in relaxing activities like deep breathing or meditation to improve your mental health. Additionally, for the sake of your mental well-being, remember to spend time with your loved ones and partake in enjoyable activities.

Long-term maintenance of your accomplishments will be easier for you to accomplish when you take care of yourself.

Here's a brief summary of the essential tactics for holding onto your successes:

Make new objectives.

Give yourself a reward. Be ready for obstacles.

Form healthy routines.

Seek assistance; remain upbeat; engage in self-care.

Recall that maintaining your accomplishments is a process rather than a final goal. Persist and never give up!

Chapter 8

Overview and health future

Honouring Your Experience
A More Robust Future

Remaining motivated and committed to your health-focused path necessitates celebrating your progress. Here are some ideas for commemorating your victories and significant anniversaries:

1. Set Milestones: Divide your objectives for wellness and health into more manageable chunks. Whether it's a goal for weight loss, fitness, or diet enhancement, acknowledge and appreciate each accomplishment.

2. Reward Yourself: Give yourself a non-food reward when you reach a goal. This could be a fun hobby, a spa day, a new fitness gadget, or a book you've been meaning to read.

3. Reflect and Journal: Consider your accomplishments and jot down your thoughts in a journal. Record your triumphs, difficulties, and emotions. It's a fantastic method to gauge your progress.

4. Share with a Support System: Tell your loved ones or friends about your accomplishments so they can encourage you on your path. Their support can be a powerful source of inspiration.

5. Before and After Photos: Take pictures of your progress to see it in visual form. It can be immensely inspiring and cause for celebration to see the changes.

6. New Wardrobe: Invest in a few new outfits that fit your healthier self as your body changes. It's a material way to honour your experience.

7. Try New Activities: Commemorate your increased level of fitness by taking up sports or new hobbies that you were previously unable to do. It's an enjoyable way to take advantage of your improved fitness and health.

8. Host a Healthy Dinner Party: Call your

loved ones over for a delectable and nutritious dinner. It's a great way to encourage others and share your new habits with them.

9. **Organise an Active Getaway**: Take an active vacation to commemorate the occasion, such as going on a bike ride or hiking in a stunning area. Enjoying your enhanced fitness in this way is gratifying.

10. **Volunteer and Give Back:** Honour the community by making a donation. Participate in events that support a cause you care about, or volunteer for a charity run.

11. **Celebrate Non-Scale Victories:** Keep in mind that there are other factors besides scale readings that affect health. Honour additional successes, such as increased vitality, restful sleep, or decreased stress.

12. Practice gratitude: Set aside some time every day to feel grateful for your body and the work you're doing to ensure your health in the future. Having gratitude can keep you inspired.

13. Set New Goals: To continue your journey and uphold your dedication to a healthier lifestyle, set new goals after you've celebrated.

Never forget that acknowledging your efforts and advancements, no matter how minor or large, is the essence of celebrating your journey. It keeps you motivated for the future and aids in reinforcing good habits. It takes a marathon, not a sprint, to maintain your accomplishments. Honour every little victory and feel pleased with your progress.

It's critical to keep in mind that you are improving every day and trying your hardest. Honour your path and have faith that you are on the correct course. You can attain your objectives and lead a healthier future if you are committed to working towards them. And remember to recognise and appreciate your progress along the way!

Finally, I would like to remind you to look after yourself. Self-care is not selfish; rather, it is essential. You can be your best self for the people and things that matter most to you if you take care of yourself. Thus, be sure to set aside some time every day for rest, relaxation, and self-care. You are deserving! And for now, that's all I have. I appreciate you coming along on this self-improvement journey with me. I hope you found this useful and educative.

One final thing, though. Recall that the objective is progress, not perfection. Avoid obsessing over the idea of being "perfect." Rather, concentrate on making advancement and acknowledging minor victories. Keep in mind that the secret to a happier and healthier life is progress rather than perfection.